The COVID Nurse Experience

My time as a nurse working with COVID patients

By Chad Newton

Copyright 2020

Acknowledgements

My thanks to the nurses and hospital workers who spoke
with me for this book. I appreciate them allowing me to
interview them about their COVID journey.

About the author

Chad Newton is a registered nurse in Philadelphia.
He's a former teacher, also in Philadelphia.
Prior to that, he worked as a television news reporter in
Syracuse, NY, and in Yonkers, NY.

March 23rd, 2020

Today, I worked in a section of the hospital here in Philadelphia that was set up for COVID patients—coronavirus disease 2019. I had three patients under my care. These were the early days of the COVID-19 infection. One patient was here to be ruled out for the disease. Her son had tested positive for COVID and she had shown some symptoms, including shortness of breath and fever. She had come to our hospital for further care.

The patient was a bit exasperated because she had gone to one hospital, had been sent home, and then had come back to us for worsening symptoms. She got a phone call from someone at the prior hospital telling her that her coronavirus test came back negative. She was itching to get out of here.

The patient demanded to speak to the doctor. The doctor explained to her that he had spoken to the prior hospital who had told him that, in fact, her COVID test was inconclusive. She was not happy to hear that she would have to wait a few more days to find out the result of our

own COVID test.

Interview with Melika Kearney, Nurse's Aide, June 23rd, 2020

Melika is a nurse's aide at a hospital in Philadelphia.

Q: I know that you got COVID… How did you find out that you had it?

Melika: "I was at work. I started feeling a little ill, like mainly, like I was having chills, slight headaches. And I was sitting down talking to a co-worker and I was telling her 'I don't feel right', and I asked her, 'Are you cold or is it just me?' And I was like, something feels a little off, and I said, 'I need to check my temperature.' So, got a thermometer, checked my temperature, it was 102.9."

She notified the manager, rechecked her temperature and called workman's comp. She had to leave to right away because fever is one of the prime COVID symptoms. She got the nasal swab done a few days later and found out that it was positive.

Q: What was your reaction when you heard that you're COVID positive?

Melika: "Now when I first took my temperature, I'm going to be honest, I cried. I cried like a baby. Just fear. Just knowing the fact, knowing how it can go. I don't have any underlying health issues or anything like that, but it was the fact that I was scared. I thought of my children, how I still had to go home. Didn't want to pass it on to them."

Q: Did you have to separate yourself from your family? Was that easy to do, hard to do?

Melika: "With my older children, it was easy because they understand that you have to stay away from mom right now. For my 6 year old, it was a little harder because he's younger, he's so affectionate, he always wants a hug, kiss, everything, so he's just like 'Mom, I can't give you a hug, I can't give you a kiss?' Like he kinda understood but not really. He's like, 'Maybe one hug a day?'"

Q: While you were home, did you have to sort of stay in the basement or in a bedroom or in some other part of the house?

Melika: "I isolated myself to the bedroom. For the most part I was mainly in the bedroom because I was mainly weak, so I couldn't really do much anyway, other than try to shower or things like that, I just stayed in the bedroom. I had my own little personal utensils, so I wouldn't use what everyone else was using."

I helped set up a unit that was set aside to eventually receive COVID patients. The floor had originally been used for seeing urology patients. There were vestiges of what the office area used to look like. There were empty desks where receptionists may have sat before to answer phone calls from patients. There was a waiting room.

The back rooms appeared to be places where patients used to be seen by the doctor. The rooms were being converted for COVID patient needs. The doors to each room were retrofitted with plastic sheeting with zippers on both sides of the door to seal the patient in and to seal others out. I imagined that as the nurse, you would have to unzip the plastic door and go inside with whatever you needed to bring to the patient, sealing yourself in.

Inside each room, there was a stretcher where the patient would eventually be. There was a machine for taking vital signs, such as blood pressure, a tool for measuring blood oxygen, as well as a thermometer. There

was a sink and there was a trash can. Those of us who

were helping set up this new COVID unit had a sinking

feeling in our stomachs about what it would be like for the

patients and the nurses who will be here.

March 30th, 2020

On this day, I was charge nurse on one of the COVID units. We had 11 patients, some designated as "rule-out" COVID, some designated as COVID positive. As charge nurse, my job was to coordinate care for all patients, making sure that rule-out patients remained isolated from each other as well as from COVID positive patients.

I assisted the nurses and aides with their work with the patients. Sometimes a nurse would go into a patient room after spending a few minutes putting an N-95 mask on, a surgical mask on top of that, a protective gown, and a face shield on top, only to find out that she forgot one medication, or the patient requests ice. My job was to be available to that nurse or aide to bring an item to them. I handed nurses ice, ice water, secondary IV tubing, an IV pump, and various medications.

It's been interesting on these COVID units. When a call light turns on, those of us who are at the nurse's station have to try to vet the calls, in order to minimize our exposure time to avoid getting infected ourselves. We are able to speak to the patient using the patient's intercom system, so we figure out what they might need and if it requires us to spend a few minutes donning protective equipment or if it's something that can be answered quickly. It's difficult when the patient is unable to project their voice loud enough over the din of the blowing negative pressure system in the room. That requires us to dress up to go in there to assist with something as simple as raising the head of the bed by a few degrees.

A few words I heard from the patients on this day: "Bless your heart", "You people are angels", "Thank you", "I know", as in "I know what you're going through".

Interview with Amanda Emmons, RN, July 8th, 2020

Amanda is a registered nurse who lives in Houston, Texas. She served as a COVID travel nurse at a hospital in the Bronx during COVID, starting on Mother's Day weekend.

Q: What was that experience like working there?

Amanda: "It was grueling, rewarding, it was gross, it was eye-opening, it was humbling, all of that; it stretched me beyond what I knew that I could possibly do. I'm just really honored that I was able to go and serve in the capacity that I was able to."

She came at a time when her agency sent out an urgent call for 500 nurses to go to New York.

Amanda: "And so, I got there and it was pretty much makeshift and just fall in line and do what you could. You know, there wasn't a whole lot of organization as it is for crisis deployment, but it was kind of scary for not only me, but the nurses around me, because we were literally walking into the belly of the beast."

Amanda worked on a medical-surgical unit where nurses helped each other get through the challenging experience.

Amanda: "It was almost like we were instant family, to make sure that everyone was covered and to make sure you felt comfortable, to help everyone in need, so I feel like I was blessed to be with the group of nurses that were placed on my unit because it was really, it was strenuous, because there were lots of codes, lots of crashes, in addition to gowning up with your personal protective equipment, going in and out of the rooms."

Amanda says they worked tirelessly in an ever-changing environment with complicated patients for 21 days straight.

Amanda: "We would leave the hotel 6 o'clock in the morning and then we would leave the hospital about 8 o'clock at night, getting back to the hotel round about 9 o'clock. I mean you know how it is, you only have time to rinse off all of the COVID, get all of that out of the way, grab something to eat, say your prayers, and go to sleep and get ready for another day."

April 2nd, 2020

I worked with a patient on a unit designated for COVID patients.   The gentleman was in his 60s and had COVID. He had diabetes, which is one of the comorbidities that coronavirus takes advantage of. He was a recent amputee (right leg above the knee).

The gentleman needed to be on 10 liters per minute of oxygen. He was pretty calm about his situation. Eventually, he was able to be weaned down to 4 liters of oxygen and we transferred him to a less intense unit.

He was replaced by a bus driver for the city transportation system. He was in his 30s and had contracted the virus by doing his job: transporting people by bus from one part of the city to another. He also had diabetes. The patient was admitted for gradually worsening shortness of breath. He came to me on 15 liters per minute of oxygen.

The interesting thing about the COVID patients is

they look like anyone else. They're just normal people

who caught a disease. They're relaxing in their beds just

like any other patient, except they have coronavirus disease

2019.

April 3rd, 2020

Today, I had a patient who was diagnosed with coronavirus. She was a woman in her 60s, who already had some problems of her own. She had a history of coronary artery disease. She had been admitted from home for acute respiratory failure. She had been intubated for a couple of days.

She was apparently on the recovery end of the disease on this day. She was on 2 liters of oxygen, had a foley catheter for urine output measurement and to protect the massive pressure ulcer wound on her sacral area of her backside. She also had a triple lumen internal jugular central line on the right side of her neck.

On this day, I removed the foley catheter to lower her risk of further infection. Also, the nurse practitioner taking care of her removed the central line from her neck, another precaution for preventing future infection.

I performed wound care with the assistance of another nurse who was taking care of the other patient in the room with my patient. We turned the patient together in order to gain access to the sacral wound. I cleaned the wound with saline and gauze. The wound was quite deep and had recently been debrided by surgeons. It bled when I wiped it with the gauze and the patient called out in pain. I encouraged her that I was almost done and it would be quick. She trembled a bit as I did the work. Then, I packed the wound with saline-soaked gauze, and finally covered up the whole thing with a foam dressing.

Interview with RN Abiola Akamo, July 1st, 2020

Abiola was stationed in the Bronx as a travel RN. She started at a time when many other travel nurses answered the call for help and worked alongside nurse practitioners and respiratory therapists whose home hospital is North Central Bronx.

Abiola: "A few of their colleagues were sick from the virus. I'm not sure if they received the PPE at the time before we arrived."

She worked on a medical-surgical unit.

Abiola: "There were enough nurses, which was extremely helpful, and there were enough supplies."

She said they had enough personal protective equipment.

Abiola: "There were times when we used surgical gowns for about a week as our protective gowns. There were times that we used the plastic, blue gowns, which is what I'm accustomed to. And then there were times when they found like the yellow mesh. But needless to say, anytime I

came into work, there were enough gowns, gloves, for sure,
there was even a time when there were enough hair nets,
shoe covers."

Abiola: "At the end they began to ration the masks, where
they were having us use it once a week. But before, it
would be about every two days, we would have a mask and
have an opportunity to change it every two days."

Q: What exactly was your reaction to having to wear an N-
95 for two days or longer?

Abiola: "For me it was a shock because when we were
fitted, the mask that they had available was the duckbill,
I'm not sure the official name. But I can't fit those. I can
only fit the 3Ms, the green ones. Small."…..

Abiola says New York's governor was adamant about
finding supplies for health care workers.

Abiola: "For wearing it one or two days, it once again was
a bit disheartening, because no one can tell you the true life
span of the mask. When we were first trained, we were all

told to have one-time use. Go into the room one time, wear the mask, and then you discard. So, to wear it for a day or two, I don't know what keeps it strong, I don't know what breaks it down. We're talking in them. We're coughing, sneezing in them."

Q: Just basically your feelings about entering the lion's den.

Abiola: "My feelings. Yes. It was definitely rocky. Rocky in the beginning when you don't know what you're getting into."

Abiola says a friend from Atlanta expressed interest in going to New York with her to work as a nurse. She said she arranged living arrangements, then the friend dropped out at the last minute.

Abiola: "You know, you don't know what you're walking into. What they had told you on the news and what I believe to be true is, you know, they're finding people dead in their homes, in the streets, as they're picking them up,

people are just coding at any age."

Abiola: "There was a moment in my kitchen where I was

shaking. And, I think, slightly hyperventilating. And I

don't have panic issues, I don't struggle with anxiety at all.

But just the weight of the decision finally sinking in. I felt

like I was a soldier going to war, being deployed. There

was a moment when I felt very patriotic. And I felt

equipped specifically for this kind of battle because I'm a

nurse and there's not that many people that could fill these

roles."

She added that one of her colleagues got sick. He was one

of the travel nurses. She ended up taking care of him as

her patient.

April 6th, 2020

I had a COVID positive patient who had been living in a nursing home. He was in his 50s, had a left above the knee amputation, and his fingers were gnarled on both hands. Some prior illness had caused his fingers to become bent into themselves: they always look like he's starting to make a fist and they don't fully extend. The patient was a hemodialysis patient who developed a fever and had to come to the hospital because the facility where he received hemodialysis refused to treat him due to his fever and the current coronavirus crisis.

I had another coronavirus patient who was in his 50s. He had a history of stroke with residual left sided weakness: almost completely paralyzed on the left side. He was able to use his right hand and move his right foot, but there was some limitation to his use of the right extremities. The patient was incontinent of bowels twice during my shift today. I had to go into the small room where he was staying and along with the nurse's aide, I was able to clean him up and give him some dignity. He lamented that he was tired of being in this condition. I encouraged him by telling him that we all get sick. He apologized to the aide and I for making a mess but we told him that it's okay.

On that same floor down the hall, there was a woman in her early 30s who had come to the hospital for shortness of breath. The doctors reported that her chest x-ray and CT scan did not show signs of COVID infection. I swabbed her nose so that the lab could check for respiratory viruses, and additionally, a special nurse came to do the COVID swab. The patient was reluctant to let the COVID swab nurse do the job, so I had to encourage her to let him do the work, just like she had let me swab her nose earlier in the day. The act of sticking a long Q-tip into someone's nostrils and moving it around is quite unpleasant for the patient. The doctors discharged her home shortly afterward because of her chest imaging and lack of deterioration, pending laboratory results.

Interview with "ABC", RN, July 8th, 2020. I changed the name to protect the nurse.

ABC is a registered nurse on a medical surgical floor at a Philadelphia hospital.

Q: Obviously you got COVID. So, how did you find out that you had it?

ABC: "I went to work. It was a Friday. Then, by the end of the shift, I was really starting to feel bad. So, I said I was going to get one of those disposable thermometers and check my temperature. Then it said 100.2. So, I said I'm going home anyway, so I'll go home and I'll take Tylenol, it must be the flu. It was still March. So, I thought, could be the flu. Never thought about COVID. Called my doctor's office the next day and told her I have the flu. She said, you may not have the flu, but you have to quarantine because you have the fever. And I said, ok, I'll quarantine. And the fever was ridiculous: it just kept going up and down. Just Tylenol and no other medication. I was in the bed for nine days. So, I took my temperature regularly, and the last one I took was 104.9 or something like that and my daughter came right away. I didn't expect her to come. I was kind of delirious at that point. They walked me out of here (home) in pajamas and a coat… and they admitted me."

She said she was admitted in a delirious and confused state. She remembers being transferred to the COVID unit as a patient and thought she was being taken to the morgue.

ABC: "And I wanted to tell the young man who was transporting me, I'm not dead. But I didn't say anything. Finally, when we were getting close to the elevator, I said, where are we going? And he was shocked to hear me say anything. You can see by his response that he was shocked that I was speaking to him. And he said, we're going to (COVID building). As long as he didn't say the morgue, I was fine."

Q: How do you think you got COVID?

ABC: "Honestly, I think I was exposed by a patient. He was a lung transplant patient and he was suspected of having COVID. Me and the PCA (Patient Care Assistant) had to transport him to the eighth floor… so they gave us all the gear and told us to gear up. And we had to tell the doctor how to gear up because he didn't know how to put the stuff on. He was putting the gown on wrong, he didn't know how to use the N95. And we did have an N95 at that time, and I was able to use it. Took him upstairs. By the time we came off the elevator, I was stripping that stuff off of me. I felt so hot. But I haven't found out if this man had COVID or not. I never got any information about him."

She remembers being in an isolation room with glass doors and hearing the doctors speaking in the hallway about her being COVID positive. She says her symptoms included being short of breath while sitting still.

Q: Did you think you were going to die?

ABC: "I definitely thought I was going to die and I told them I wanted to be DNR (Do Not Resuscitate). I did not want to be intubated, I didn't want to go on any machine. I just didn't want to do that. I didn't want to have that experience. I didn't want them to do that to my body."

A nurse that she knows came and took off the DNR bracelet and said, 'we're not going to let you be DNR'. The nurse encouraged her that she wasn't going to die and she'd be back to work soon.

Q: Now that you've been through it, do you place any blame on any entity or any situation for the fact that you got COVID?

ABC: "I don't want to say blame but I want to say mismanagement. Because you knew. They knew that this disease was out there and they should have protected us prior to being exposed. We should have been protected."

Q: You don't think we were protected early enough?

ABC: "No, because the only reason why I wore a mask in any of the patients' rooms at that time was if they were transplant patients. For the rest of the patients, we were unmasked. We had masks, but we weren't told to wear them. We didn't know that we were being exposed to anything because it was new. And the people who knew what the disease progression would be, they knew about China. I'm not from China; I didn't experience anyone from China, or I didn't leave the country, so I thought I was safe, because I was at work."

She thought she would never leave the hospital alive.

ABC: "It was a horrible experience that no one should have to go through that, the way it happened. I shouldn't have been made to stay home all those days, suffering, when I could have really lost my life in my own bed, because they kept saying, oh just self-quarantine. But they weren't saying that you may have COVID or let's test you. No one even tested me until I got to the hospital. I should have been tested when I told my doctor I had this fever. And she

suspected it, but she never said let's test to confirm it."

April 7th, 2020

We've been overwhelmed by the support from the community around us here in Philadelphia. For many days now, since the COVID outbreak started unfolding, we've been hearing in some way from our community. After the city shut down all non-essential businesses, people were looking for ways to contribute. What it turned into for those of us who work on the hospital floors, is food.

Every day we get tons of food from various organizations and restaurants. Yesterday, we received a box of some of the tastiest pastries. Small, multi-layer cakes, tiny cinnamon buns, small slices of blueberry bagels. That came with coffee and creamer and sugar. Today, we received individually wrapped lunches from a well-known area deli. Each box contained a sandwich made with tuna, turkey or cheese, along with a bag of chips and a cookie. They also sent us drinks such as iced tea, as well as athletic-type brand name beverages that you would find on the sidelines of a national sporting event.

The notes were the best part. Hand-written notes said things such as: "Superman has nothing on you." "Thanks for being a hero." "Thank you for your services." "You are my hero." "Thank you for saving lives." "You're my hero!" Those notes made me pause and cry. And I shared my crying with my colleagues. And we agreed that it's okay to cry. We must pour out our hearts so that we can put our face masks back on and put our face shields back on and put our protective gowns back on so we can go take care of our COVID patients.

April 11th, 2020

It's the weekend, but we still have to work. As
nurses, many of us have to work some weekends each
month. In my current job, I work every other weekend. At
a prior job, I worked every third weekend. It's interesting
walking into the hospital building that's been designated
for COVID patients. When you enter the double doors,
there are three people waiting, each armed with a hand-held
forehead scanning thermometer to check our temperatures.
The machine beeps and you're allowed into the building, or
your flagged and turned away if you have a fever.

Further into the lobby of this building, you see
that it's been transformed. A temporary wall has been set
up with a temporary "door", which is no more than sheets
of hard plastic that a person would have to walk through to
enter what has become a holding area for COVID patients.
Once flagged as "possible COVID" by the emergency
department, some of the patients are sent to this area.
There are beds side by side in the lobby, away from the

eyes of passersby, behind the temporary wall. I never worked in this lobby, but I've spoken to other nurses who have.

Also, in this lobby, there are people who check for your name against a list of names they were given by the people who staff the hospital. They double check to see which floor you're supposed to report to. At the same time, they give you an N-95 mask. They also ask if you still have your face shield that was given to you prior. The face shield is meant to stop droplets from COVID from entering your eyes. The N-95 mask is supposed to stop droplets from entering your nose or mouth.

Interview with DEF, RN, July 9th, 2020. I changed the name to protect the nurse.

DEF works at a long-term acute care facility (LTAC) in the suburbs of Philadelphia.

Q: What has it been like for you working with COVID patients over the past couple of months.

DEF: "Honestly, it's been scary. Normally, you go in to work and you are mindful that, yes, your patient can crash and, yes, you are here to be the nurse and you are here to protect them. Not protect essentially but do the best you can to make sure that they are safe and you can more or less keep them alive. Because that's really our goal. But now you're thinking of 'I'm putting myself in harm, I'm putting my loved ones in harm', so it's another layer of stress that's an already a chaotic job at times."

Q: They've been testing the patients?

DEF: "They have been. They've been very aggressive. Initially, they were kind of hesitant. We actually didn't have any COVID patients but then, I think, what happened was, there was a staff member who had COVID and one patient got infected, and then I think a couple of patients said they were under their care, got tested and then one of them actually was positive for COVID. So that's how COVID came into our doors."

Q: What was it like when people found out that one of the staff members had COVID?

DEF: "Oh my God, it was surreal because, I think, even though we were seeing, we were hearing it on the news, it just became more of a reality, it just became more serious. Even though it's like, yes we know that we come here, especially, you are putting yourself on the line, even pre-COVID, you're putting yourself on the line, you're putting your life on the line, but now it's just like, it really affirms, I'm putting my health at risk. And, also, it just reaffirms that this is like the real deal. It's a real war. A real health war."

Q: What are your feelings about seeing COVID coming back stronger in other states?

DEF: "I think leadership a hundred percent factors into how much people will assume responsibilities for themselves. Because all throughout when you're watching the news, they talk about how this is a public health crisis, so it's not just a matter of doctors and nurses who are responsible for their patients. It's also about individuals being responsible for themselves, be responsible for

their families, be responsible for their neighbors. So, it's the job of general public to kind of like come together and fight this virus."

April 12th, 2020

Looking at the four patients in my care this weekend, I see a pattern. They're all COVID positive, yes, but all of them have two similar underlying health conditions: diabetes and high blood pressure. I had a man in his 30s, a woman in her 40s, a man in his 60s, and a man in his 70s, and they each have diabetes and high blood pressure. Scientists and doctors have mentioned that people with certain underlying health problems, such as diabetes, lung problems and heart problems are more susceptible to COVID.

One of the patients was ready to go home: the man in his 30s. I received him on 2 liters per minute of oxygen. I conducted an ambulatory pulse oximetry test with him, during which I turned off his oxygen, walked with him for 200 feet while checking his blood oxygen saturation using a device. His heart rate increased slightly, he was slightly short of breath, but he did not desaturate below 90%. He looked good, like a normal, average guy in his 30s. He couldn't go home yet, however, because he lives with two people who would also be especially susceptible to COVID. The case management team has been working to find him placement at a local hotel until he is completely cleared of the virus.

The man in his 70s was also on room air. The gentleman was ready to go home. His discharge has been complicated by his self-care deficit. His wife died of COVID and he is unable to take care of himself alone. His children live far away. The case management team has been attempting to find a place for him, however, in light of his COVID infection, it's especially hard to place him. Facilities that normally accept people his age are not accepting them because of his COVID infection. COVID has been raging through nursing homes and killing patients.

This gentleman could not go home on his own. During the night one day, he dressed himself in his home clothes and attempted to leave the hospital, much to the chagrin of the night shift nurse. I worked with him the next day. I had to dress him up in the hospital gown after removing his wet home clothes and cleaning him. He had been incontinent of urine. I found a reclining chair to place next to his bed so that he could have a good place to sit. I locked the wheels of the chair so that he didn't fall. I placed a pad on the chair to catch his urine for the next episode of incontinence. He asked me if I liked jazz music, and although I'm not necessarily a fan, I was able to find some jazz on YouTube on the computer in his room and I left that playing for him. This made his day.

The woman in her 40s was discharged this weekend. She was quite ambulatory while I took care of her. She was thrilled when I brought her discharge paperwork. I had to give her some instruction and teaching on checking her blood sugar and administering insulin.

Before this hospitalization, she had been taking metformin pills at home to control her blood sugar. During the day, I demonstrated for her how to check her blood sugar. I also asked her to demonstrate back to me how to check her blood sugar. When her home insulin came from

the pharmacy, I showed her how to draw up insulin from

the vial. I asked her to then demonstrate back to me how to

do it.

I gave her a stern warning about the effects too

much insulin can have on her body. I informed her of the

side effects of low blood sugar. I also told her that she

should teach someone else in her household how to check

her blood sugar, in case she becomes incapacitated due to

low blood sugar from an insulin overdose. I told her that if

her blood sugar drops below 50 that she should call 911 for

help.

April 16th, 2020

On this day, I was moved to the intensive care setting. Just as I had predicted, the number of critically ill patients is increasing. The hospital has expanded its ICU capabilities to accommodate the growing number of patients. We were asked to go to a section of the hospital that's normally an operating room area. There, we were paired up with ICU nurses and worked together to take care of patients on ventilators.

The patients were in negative pressure rooms, where the air is sucked into the room when the door opens. This keeps the contaminated air within the patient's room. The ventilated patients looked quite sick. All of them were in various stages of sedation to prevent them from pulling at their tubes. Some were newly ventilated, with breathing tubes placed into their mouths. Others already had a tracheostomy placed into the middle of the front of their necks.

Today, I spent some time familiarizing myself
with the ICU setting. I've been a medical surgical nurse
for several years but have never worked in an ICU.
Usually in the ICU, nurses work with two patients due to
their acuity level. ICU patients are the sickest patients,
therefore they need more attention. Medical surgical
nurses usually have 4-6 patients, depending on where you
work. Med surg patients are not as sick as ICU patients. I
spent some time getting the lay of the land, to figure out
where supplies were kept. We were all trying to become
familiar, from nurses to doctors to aides, because none of
us usually works in the operating room setting, which is
where we found ourselves today.

Interview with Maria Pasion, ICU RN, July 9th, 2020

Maria works at a hospital in the suburbs of New York City. She said the COVID experience has been like a roller coaster, due to not knowing what would happen next. The months of March, April, and May were an experience like she's never had before.

Q: How come you think we were unprepared?

Maria: "Even though you hear that from the media, we never, especially because it's in New York, we were hit the hardest. We never thought that we would run out of supplies, because at one point we did. That's when I could say that we were unprepared. Ventilators, that's true, at one point we ran out of it. At one point we ran out of just basic supplies to care for the patient, and most especially the PPE (personal protective equipment)."

Q: How scary was that?

Maria: "It was very scary because they tell you something different every day. And everybody is doing their best.

Doctors, the researchers in the news, the nurses, everybody

is doing their best, but it's a new thing. Even though we

take care of flu, we take care of tuberculosis… Our ICU

was overrun and we had to open up new ICUs. We tripled

our capacity so that's scary."

Q: What was that like having to handle critically ill COVID

patients?

Maria: "Normally in the ICU when you have somebody

who is very, very critical, you will be one-to-one with that

patient. And oftentimes, when you're staffed very well,

you will have two nurses with that one patient. It came to a

point where we would have two or three of them, very

critical care patients and you have less staff, and we were

asking for help from the step-down floors. The step-down

nurses stepped up and helped us, but they're not trained for

that so we were also mentoring them and taking care of our

critical patients ourselves. It was overwhelming."

Q: Do you think it was a little too much for the ICU nurses to handle such critical patients by themselves for such an extended period of time?

Maria: "Absolutely, because, like I said, we would have one critical care patient, like very, very critical, in our unit, which is an eight-bed unit. We have two ICUs, so 16 beds. But then you'll have the rest of the unit will be stable critical care patients who would go out of the ICU and go to the step-down floor after three, four days and they'll be walking again. Not all of them but I would say, a lot of them are, because there'll be surgical ICU patients. They're there for closer monitoring and then they go. But this, they stayed, and they died. Some of them instantly, some of them lingered for weeks. Very critical. You would think at one point they would take a turn and be okay, but then they'll come back, or they'll have another complication, and it was on and on and on and it went on for three months with all these COVID patients. And it was very overwhelming."

April 17th, 2020

Today I spent some time getting to know the patients under my care. One of them had some good news today. She's a woman in her 30s, who was successfully taken off the ventilator. They had been giving her ventilator breathing at night, but last night for the first time, she didn't need it to maintain proper oxygenation. She even asked for a chair so she could get out of bed. She was attached to oxygen via a trach collar, which is basically a tube with an opening at the end where oxygen blows into the tracheostomy opening in her neck. It was with great pleasure that I found her a nice recliner chair so she could sit down and not be confined to the bed. I also got her a bedside commode so that when she needed it, she could use it instead of the bedpan. Small steps matter.

We were getting phone calls from the people who manage patient movement, telling us that we needed to accept a few more ventilated patients. Those of us on the receiving end realized that the grim reality was setting in. More sick patients were coming.

I went with my partner ICU nurse to another floor to pick up one of those patients. She was attached to a ventilator as well as an IV pole with several drips running. In order to move her from that floor to the modified operating room where we were heading, we needed two people to maneuver the bed, one person to push the IV pole, another person to push the ventilator, while the respiratory therapist handled the transport breathing machine. Four nurses and a respiratory therapist made this move happen. The patient had to be monitored the entire time to make sure nothing else went wrong.

April 20th, 2020

I returned to work to find an empty bed where my patient once was. I found out by speaking to my colleague that he had died over the past few days. The gentleman had succumbed to his COVID illness. My colleague was not sure exactly what went wrong. He had died over the weekend. They attempted to save him by doing CPR, but it didn't work. During the day, I found a sticky note that someone had posted on a computer at the nurse's station. It had his wife's name and phone number.

This was a real person with real family who had lost him. And they were not there to see him at the end. The nature of the COVID illness triggered some new hospital policies around the country and the world, which included that patients' family members were not allowed to come into the hospital to visit them, except for end of life situations. Despite that caveat, it happened so quickly for this gentleman that his family didn't have an opportunity to come say goodbye.

There was some hope during this same day. One of the patients I took care of in the previous few days was discharged. The case management and social work team found an appropriate long-term care setting for her. She was elated to hear the news first thing in the morning that she would be getting out of this COVID environment. I imagine that she had some personal trauma to deal with in the next few months of her life after living through COVID. A crew came to pick her up with a stretcher. They were wearing full white body suits and masks. She herself had to wear a mask to protect others upon her departure. It was good seeing her leave the hospital alive and on her way to recovery.

April 21ˢᵗ, 2020

Today I reflect on a conversation I had with a colleague about her father. He lived in a southern U.S. city and contracted COVID. My colleague works in another department at my hospital. She came to the floor where I was working and just happened to pull me aside to ask me some questions about the COVID patients. I had never met her before, but she just watched the floor for a little while, listening to us talking, and then she started a conversation with me.

Her father had been on a ventilator and the family decided that they didn't want him to live like this anymore. My colleague asked me about some of the comorbidities that I've seen in COVID patients, and I mentioned diabetes and hypertension. She said he had those two diseases as well. What especially concerned her was that his diabetes and hypertension were under control. He had been taking his medications as far as she knew.

Her story is the story of many other people who were now facing this killer epidemic. Lives were being turned upside down. COVID was sweeping across the land, infecting people one at a time. Some people got mild symptoms from the illness but others

ended up in hospitals, on oxygen, on ventilators, and some died, including my colleague's father.

April 24, 2020

It's quite interesting what we've had to wear to protect ourselves from the novel coronavirus. And the steps we have to take throughout the nursing day to keep ourselves as clean as possible. From the moment we walk into the building, someone takes our temperature by pointing a thermometer at our heads.   It looks like a gun and the person pointing it looks like the executioner. Thankfully, my temperature has been running normal.

When entering our work areas after finding out which floor we're assigned to for the day, we get the feeling that we're entering a place that's infected. Based on what we know so far as of this writing, the coronavirus enters our body through the nose, eyes and mouth. They give us an N-95 respirator mask for use for the day. In the past, I remember, N-95s were used once to enter an infected patient's room and thrown out when leaving the patient's room.

We protect our eyes with a face shield. It's a long,

plastic shield that covers your face from the forehead down

to below the chin. It's supposed to prevent droplets of

coronavirus from splashing into our faces.

Some people have been wearing a regular surgical

mask on top of the N-95 mask. The surgical mask is meant

to catch the droplets that would have hit the N-95.

Theoretically, people would then toss out the surgical mask

after going into each patient's room. But there are not

enough surgical masks to maintain that luxury. As a result,

people have been wearing the surgical mask on top of the

N-95 mask all day long. But not everyone has done that.

Some people have been wearing just the N-95.

We've also had the luxury of head covers. The

hospital has provided us with hair nettings to cover our

hair. And we have disposable gowns that we wear on top

of our scrubs. By the time we're fully protected, we look

like we belong in a movie about a worldwide pandemic.

But of course, we're living that movie.

You should see us when it's time to eat. We go through elaborate processes to remove our protective equipment. First, we place a paper towel on a surface. Then we carefully reach behind our head to either remove the face shield or to point it further up. Next we reach behind our ears to find the strings of the masks, which we then gingerly place on top of the paper towel, while hoping that a little coronavirus doesn't get loose and find a happy place to grow in one of us. Then we wash our hands and we eat.

We've had some discussion among ourselves about how lucky we are. We're lucky that after working in a coronavirus environment for weeks straight, most of us have not become infected apparently. Some of the staff have had to take some time off. I heard about other nurses who have to be in quarantine for various reasons. Others have come down with fever or cough. Others have tested positive for the virus and have had to stay home.

As the days go by and you enter patient room after patient room, you develop this steel determination within you. Coronavirus or CDIF or flu or ESBL or MRSA, we're healthcare workers. This one is new but it's slowly becoming less novel. We dress up for battle and we go in. There is this mild panic when you're in a patient's room and they cough. You hope and pray that the face shield blocks the little droplets, and if they're light enough to blow around the face shield, that the mask will catch them in the fibers, and if the little droplets get on your gown, that when you leave the room and you take the gown off, the little droplets will only have themselves to play with in the trash can. And that when you wash your hands, they'll slip off into the sink and go play with each other in the city's drainage system, away from us.

Some of us have talked about the futility of our actions. We know from education that we're supposed to protect ourselves from the virus using handwashing, gloves, mask, gown and face shield. But from talking to experienced nurses around me, we realize that this virus is

powerful. It's designed so well that it can get around many

of our protections. All it requires is one slip-up. You

might protect yourself quite well, but if the person next to

you waffles a bit, the virus uses that opportunity.

Doorknobs really make you think nowadays. Faucets, light

switches, railings, chairs, tables and elevator buttons all

make you think. What's sitting on there? That's why some

of us look at it as futility. What's the adverse effect of

using so many chemicals to clean surfaces? What does it

do to our skin? What's in the chemicals? What does that

do to our immune system over time? Although we

continue to protect ourselves based on the

recommendations of scientists, we also know that we have

to balance one thing with another.

Public health officials have propagated

information about flattening the curve. The curve is the

rate of infection for a particular area. Different states have

been doing daily news conferences, putting out information

about the date and the number of infections. Each day you see the curve steepen. Their point is that if we stay home then we will give the virus fewer opportunities to transmit from person to person. The more we social distance, the slower the rate of infection. Therefore, the curve will flatten.

But people have become restless. Weeks into the pandemic, people are itching to get out of their homes. It's spring, the weather is becoming more pleasant, the grass is growing on the lawns, the flowers are blooming, the trees are becoming green. People want to go back to their way of living before the coronavirus plagued us. There are quite a few people who want to stay indoors because they're worried that they'll become victim to the virus. But there are many others who are itching to get back out there.

Slowly, I see more people gathering in small groups on the corners. Some are tossing dice against buildings in small groups. Some are smoking cigarettes with their pals. Some are sharing bags of chips and soda.

Few places are open now, other than essential businesses,

and on warmer days, I go running in the woods. One day I

saw so many people in the park that I felt unsafe. I felt like

the virus had plenty of opportunities to spread in this park

where people were doing something that would normally

be considered healthy: exercising. But there were too

many of us exercising in the same place, and each of us

could potentially become a vector (or carrier) for the virus.

One person coughs, another person breathes in or the virus

can land on the eyeball and boom, you have a spread.

What a nightmare.

April 27th, 2020

Even the nurses are getting frustrated. Today, we had some discussion about how it would be great to just get back to normal. We miss our former unit where we worked before the coronavirus disease hit our area. I took a look at some of us today and I wondered "how did we get to this?" We were sitting at the computers documenting on our patients, but we're all wearing protective equipment. Head covers, masks, face shields and gowns. I remarked, who would have thought months ago that we would all be sitting here looking like we're about to go welding or fight off some horrific infectious disease? In fact, one nurse was wearing a protective shield that was fashioned after a welder's helmet.

Today it seemed that some our more able COVID patients did not want to stay in the hospital. Several people left against medical advice. One of my patients was a bit rowdy from the beginning of the day. The diabetic demanded syrup for his pancakes several times while I was in his room wearing full protective gear. I assured him

each time that I would go look for syrup for him when I got

out of the room.

It's quite an elaborate process going in and out of

these rooms. The converted room is sealed with a zip-up

door. The temporary plastic door has zippers on both sides,

so when you go in our out, you zip yourself in or your zip

yourself out. I eventually found this gentleman some

sugar-free syrup.

Not long after, while I was in another location,

people came to me telling me that my patient is in the

hallway threatening to leave. I dropped what I was doing

and indeed, there was my patient, dressed in street clothes,

ready to go. I attempted to coax him back to his room, but

he was shaking his head "no". I had gauze and tape in my

hands because I've seen this before, so I proceeded to

remove the IV access line in his left arm, with his

permission. I applied pressure for a little while and then I

put tape on it.

The gentleman was rearing to go, even after I asked him to wait while I call the doctor. As he was proceeding toward the exit, I saw a trail of blood. I knew it was from the IV site. I stopped him and told him "you're bleeding". I used more gauze to apply pressure and held it hard, all the while calling other nurses to come help me. "Go get gauze," I said. The chaotic scene got more chaotic with the man shouting that he's leaving and that he's not staying. Of course, his mask was halfway down his face. Thankfully, all of us near him had on our protective equipment.

I escorted the gentleman to the main lobby after I fixed his mask. Only after he walked out was I able to call the doctor to let him know that the patient eloped. If a person is of sound mind and we don't have a physician's order to hold him (such as a psychiatric 302 order), we can't hold him. He has a right as a person to be free. Off he went into the world with COVID and a dialysis catheter in his right chest wall, to do God knows what.

April 29th, 2020

Face masks

One of the most spectacular novelties that has come from COVID is face masks. Home-made face masks are making appearances everywhere. They range in all types of colors, shapes and sizes. It started with people just wrapping bandanas around their faces. Then it turned into a more skilled operation, with some folks taking that same bandana and shaping it up or their faces, and also attaching strings or elastic.

Some of us nurses have received home-made face masks as gifts. During the workday, people have brought us various types of masks that they made themselves and the masks have been distributed to staff members. Some have pleats in the front like louvers. Others are flat straight across. Some have a slight up-curve for the nose.

The attachments vary as well. In some masks, the elastic is attached four times near each corner. Others have an opening for elastic across the top and across the bottom

of the masks and then the elastic gets looped on top of the

nose and under the chin. Some masks have openings on

the left and right side, where the elastic gets threaded

through and then gets looped around the ears.

I think people are embracing masks because

they've become a necessity and you can be creative with

them. People have shown up with fabric masks made of

Disney characters. Others display African themes,

sunshine, clouds, the sky, trees, the ocean. You name it,

there's a mask like that. And there's a mask for the

conservative person who likes plain colors, as well as for

the colorful person looking to make a statement.

I started making masks on my sewing machine

just to wear to the grocery store. I put a couple of those

first masks on Facebook and the response was incredible.

People were asking me to send them a mask or two. I

started a small business and we will see where it goes. I

ship the masks to people around the United States using the

post office. I also started making matching head-hands,

head-wraps and wristbands.

April 30th, 2020

Today I worked on one of the units that I helped
set up at the beginning of the coronavirus crisis. It was the
unit that had been used for urology offices before COVID-
19 hit. This is the unit with the zip-up plastic doors with
red tape to seal the plastic on the door frames. I had four
patients today, each with positive COVID swabs or chest
imaging that made them highly probable COVID positive.

The news today is that part of the unit would be
closing down. The unit was spread around the 6th floor of
this building. Half of it was set to close today. Patients on
the closing side would be moved to the side where I was
working. I asked my manager if there were fewer COVID
patients and without actually answering, he crossed his
fingers and had a look of hope from behind his mask as he
shrugged.

We were all sharing that hope as we talked that
day. Many of us expressed our frustration with COVID
and how we're ready to go back to normal. We personified

COVID and said things like, "You've proven to us what you can do, now get out of here."

We got food today from a well-known fast-food restaurant. The chicken sandwiches came in pretty, white boxes. There was a bag of chips in there, too, as well as a cookie. We devoured the salty treats, knowing full well this is not how we normally eat. But there is something about comfort food during times of crisis. You don't feel guilty about it. You just eat and savor. And you look forward to more the next time.

I had a screaming, bipolar, schizophrenic patient who drove me bananas today. He kept pushing his call light button to ask for medications that I had already given him and also to ask for medications that he had looked up on the internet. Staff kept taking turns to answer his requests.

At the end of the shift he demanded metoprolol, which is a heart rate and blood pressure medication. He kept looking at his monitor, which was showing a slightly elevated heart rate. But the interesting thing is, as the

minutes passed, his heart rate kept going up. I tried

explaining to him that he is making his heart rate go up by

agitating himself.

He threatened to leave, kept talking about atrial

fibrillation, said how he knows his body, called the

emergency department to complain about us, said we were

doing "nothing" for him and he wants a wheelchair to

leave. Fortunately, 7 pm came and it was time for

nightshift, but I gave him the scheduled 8 pm metoprolol

just a little after 7, to pave the way for a little peace for my

nightshift colleague who would be inheriting him.

May 1st, 2020

I was back on the 4th floor today, which had become my new home during this COVID crisis. The first thing I noticed upon arriving there is that they had already closed off half of the floor. There had been patients in the wide-open waiting room of that floor. There had been beds lined up next to each other with patients separated by curtains placed on stands. But those patients were not there anymore. They had been moved or discharged home.

It was interesting walking through that section today. The converted space had many of the necessities of health care, except there were no people. There were beds, there were IV poles with IV pumps on them, there were monitors for heart rate, heart rhythm and blood oxygenation. The carpeted flooring was covered in a double layer of thick plastic. There was a nurse's station, where I imagine a secretary or two used to sit to greet patients and get them organized to see other staff.

The makeshift COVID unit had supplies stowed away in corners. Blankets, sheets, socks, patient gowns, chuck pads for beds, blood pressure cuffs, thermometers, IV bags from dextrose to saline, IV tubing, piggyback tubing, IV needles, IV start kits, gauze, tape and gloves. You could run a small community hospital with the stuff we had here on this floor. But we always needed more supplies as the day went by.

The morning medication pass has become so intense that doctors have scheduled medications for 8 a.m. instead of the normal 10 a.m. It takes us nurses so long to prepare the medications because of the extra garb that we have to wear. Also, medications are located in several different places on the floor, not just in one machine. And sometimes, the medications are not on the floor, so we have to request them from the pharmacy. I imagine that the pharmacy itself has had to scramble to accommodate the new COVID demands while still servicing the rest of the non-COVID hospital.

Many patients get IV antibiotics, especially

ceftriaxone. I had to set up a system where once the IV

antibiotic is finished infusing, the IV pump would switch to

what we call a KVO (keep vein open), which is 5-10mL an

hour of saline. This buys me time because the pump won't

beep after the antibiotic is finished. Of course, that takes

time to set up.

It was a logistical nightmare to accomplish every

morning, but it was necessary because after I was finished

with one patient, I would then go on to the next patient and

not have to worry about the IV pump beeping. But each

patient required about a half hour of my time the first time I

saw them in the morning. They may have pain that needs

to be addressed, they may have toileting needs, there may

be full trash cans. Primarily only nurses went into these

rooms, so we had to do the work of housekeeping in

addition to our regular nursing duties.

May 4th, 2020

Hair Covers

We had a conversation today about the different head-wraps and hats that people have been wearing lately. COVID-19 is a sticky virus that hangs in the air, and we've been protecting ourselves with head gear as well. The hospital has been giving us hair netting but we've also been coming up with our own designs.

Nurses have been looking up tutorial videos on the web to figure out the best ways to make head gear. Some have come up with interesting designs. One nurse created something that looks like it came out of a story book. It's a bonnet that ties in the back. It's tied tightly around the forehead but becomes fluffy as it leaves the forehead.

Another nurse came up with a design that's like a surgical cap but in cloth. It's one consistent piece that goes around the front and sides of the head to meet in the back, and on top of the head there's a piece of cloth to cover the hair. Strings bring it all together in the back.

My design was more of a head-wrap. I've come up with two different types of head-wraps. I find that the longest part of the creation is the hemming. It takes me a whole hour to make one. My design features a flat piece of cloth about 15 inches long with four ends. All the edges have to be hemmed so that the fabric stays together. Whoever uses it just ties each of the four ends at the back to secure the hair in there.

COVID, in my world, is not going away. Today I worked on a converted PACU unit (Post Anesthesia Care). Normally, patients here would be post-surgical as they start recovering. This unit was converted to a COVID unit. Temporary walls were set up to separate the patients where curtains used to be. Between every two rooms there was an anteroom set up. Plastic doors with zippers were set up here. You zip yourself into the anteroom and then you zip yourself into the patient's room on the right or the patient's room on the left.

My colleague told me about her COVID patients that she had today. Somehow, she got two patients who also had family members in the hospital. One man was a dialysis patient whose wife was on another floor with COVID as well. And another man was on high flow oxygen and his wife was in the ICU. This particular ICU patient happened to be a nurse. The gentleman was to be transferred to the same ICU where his wife is because his condition was deteriorating in terms of his oxygen needs. Their rooms would be close to each other.

It was sobering to hear that a nurse had caught COVID and that her husband had it too. When you hear news like that, you think it could happen to anyone. We work in COVID every day at this point and it's only a matter of time before we ourselves possibly get COVID. But we come to work.

There were some nurses from my floor who I had not seen for a week or two. Word had gotten around that so-and-so may have COVID. When they came back to work, I asked them what happened and they told me that they had symptoms suggesting COVID and had self-quarantined. Some had tested positive for COVID. It's incredible to think that this scary virus was working its way through the ranks of the nurses. What can you do? You go to work, you wear your personal protective equipment, and you wash your hands. And you hope that you don't get sick.

May 10th, 2020

I spoke to a seasoned registered nurse today about our experience with COVID so far. She reminisced about the day that she first came to the COVID building that we've been working in. She's seen many things in her many years of nursing, but this was overwhelming for her.

To give you some background, the building that we're working in is across the street from the rest of the hospital where we normally work and it is connected by a covered bridge. She said when she stood at one end of the bridge that first day, the thought that flashed in her mind was, "Yeah though I walk through the valley of the shadow of death, I will fear no evil." She said at the time, the bridge looked so long and she looked at it as 'the last mile'. But she walked, accompanied by another nurse.

This experienced nurse reflected that she had quite a reaction to coming toward the COVID building. She said her palms were sweaty and her heart was racing. But her years of steel kicked in. She discussed one particular

COVID unit which was wide open, with patient beds side by side, men and women separated by a mere curtain tied to two poles, and the floor was covered in plastic sheeting, and the high-flow oxygen was blowing

COVID all over the place, and we had masks on and face shields and gowns to protect us, but we were in the middle of this thing. Despite her fears, she decided to pull up her britches, tighten her belt and get to work.

I discharged a woman in her 50s today. I asked her how she caught COVID and she said she works in a place for senior citizens. She told me she's the only one in her family who got infected, so I gave her a little advice in conjunction with CDC guidelines: remain in your private space for two weeks, wear a mask when around others, ask your family to bring you food at your bedroom door, stay six feet away from others.

I had a patient in her 80s today. She had come to the hospital with shortness of breath and had fallen at home. The night-shift nurse who passed her to me said that overnight she had been requiring more oxygen. The patient

was on room air at the beginning of the night shift but by

the end of the 12-hour shift, she was on 3 liters of oxygen

because her oxygen saturation was dropping below 90%.

A good oxygen saturation is 95% and up.

That morning, I noticed right away that the

woman looked a little ashen in her face. I gave her the

morning antibiotics, including ceftriaxone and

azithromycin. Her oxygen level was only 90%, so I

bumped her up to 5 L. On this particular unit where I'm

stationed today, that is the maximum amount of oxygen we

can give. I decided to monitor the patient for a while, to

see what happens. She was not short of breath and she was

not in distress. Calm and beautiful in her 80s.

But after a few hours, her oxygen level continued

to drop to the upper 80s and I decided to notify the doctor.

Later, I transferred the patient to another floor that can

provide more oxygen. It was sad to see her go, because

she's someone's grandmother or great-grandmother. I hoped that she would recover as I said goodbye to her.

I later admitted a woman in her 20s who also had shortness of breath and fatigue. She was a COVID rule-out, meaning she would be admitted to this floor until testing came back to say 'yes' or 'no'. Her CT scan and X-ray showed what looked like COVID (ground glass opacity) so she was sent to my floor. She too got a dose of ceftriaxone and azithromycin from me as soon as she arrived.

A gentleman that I treated today was quite a challenge for us. He refused medications from the night-shift nurse and chased her out of the room to the point where she feared for her safety. I was a bit concerned about going into the room. He was recently diagnosed with kidney failure and had recently been started on dialysis and he apparently had some psychiatric problems as well.

When I entered his room with the blood sugar machine and his pills, I introduced myself as his nurse and attempted to gauge who I'd be dealing with for the 12-hour

shift. Within seconds he told me he was getting out of here

today and, as far as the doctors, he uttered a few expletives.

I documented verbatim what he said to me. I told him he

has a right to leave as an adult. I also told him I'd be

informing the doctors about his plans to leave. He refused

all medications, including his kidney and blood pressure

medications. But he did allow me to check his blood sugar,

I did his vitals signs (blood pressure, temperature, heart

rate, respiratory rate), and he allowed me to do an

assessment using a stethoscope. I breathed a sigh of relief

that he was not that bad.

The doctor came to see him and helped him

understand that the reason he should not leave the hospital

against medical advice is that there are few dialysis

facilities that can accommodate COVID patients. He

informed the patient that case management and social work

had been looking for places for him where he can get

dialysis near his house, as opposed to far from home.

The patient's attitude teetered from cooperation to defiance throughout the day, but he did not leave against medical advice. He allowed me to administer insulin at lunchtime. At dinner, he refused to let me check his blood sugar or vital signs. It was just one big "no" in that room by the end of the shift.

I checked on the computer system today and saw that a patient I had worked with in the ICU a few weeks ago had died. She had been in critical condition for a while, on a ventilator, and had been receiving many drips to keep her alive. I recognized the name in the deceased list, had a few reflective thoughts, and I sent a few feelings through the air to her family who had to deal with her loss. Such is the nature of COVID.

May 11th, 2020

Word has been spreading via Whatsapp that our
unit where we normally work might be reopening soon.
Someone who works on our floor started a group chat with
us. I suppose the benefit of the group chat is to keep us
informed about what's going on around the hospital,
because we're so disjointed right now. Some days you see
your colleagues if you're lucky enough to work with them
on the same COVID floor, and other days you don't see
people for weeks and you wonder if something happened to
them.

Apparently, they're reopening our old unit this
week. Slowly at first, is what I heard. Half the beds will
be occupied and the other half will remain empty. I feel
odd about it, and I'm not sure why. I feel like COVID is
not over yet so I'm wondering why they're shifting us back
over there. I did meet some newly hired nurses on the
COVID units recently. It's possible that the hospital is
bringing in the new hires to handle the COVID needs. I

feel for these new nurses, though, because they're not only

new to the hospital, they're also new to COVID. Imagine

having to familiarize yourself with a new facility while

handling COVID patients.

I did speak to one of the new nurses a few days

ago while I was working with her. She asked typical

questions such as where we keep certain supplies. Also,

she was a bit frustrated by her patient load because she had

two screaming patients. Can you imagine you're getting

orientation for one day as a pool nurse and then you're

thrown into the COVID zone? I suppose they knew what

they were signing up for but it seems a bit too much to

handle. But that is the nature of nursing sometimes.

People have called us heroes. People have called

us "superman". But what I've been saying is we're just

doing our duty. This is our job. We did sign up to do this.

When I was a special education teacher, I knew that I had

to go into the classroom and teach students that had

difficulty learning. It was not an easy job but it was a

rewarding job. I did it for more than 7 years. As a nurse, I
report for duty. Prison guards have to go to work in the
prison. That's their job. Firefighters run into burning
buildings. That's their job. Police officers sometimes run
into dark alleys at night chasing after criminals with guns.
We report for duty.

May 14, 2020

As the rumors had said, our unit is back open.
Today, we arrived at our building and headed straight to
our pre-COVID floor. Still, just as a reminder that it ain't
over till it's over, a person was standing at the entrance to
the regular building with a thermometer to check our
temperatures on our foreheads. And, she was giving out
surgical masks for staff to wear all day.

The differences were stark, however. When we
got to our floor, there were many familiar smiling faces
welcoming us back. Some of those we had not seen in a
few weeks were those who were not able to go to the
COVID floors for various reasons, including underlying
health conditions that would have made them vulnerable to
the virus. Gone were the temporary, plastic doors with
zippers and red tape. Gone were the gowns that we had to
wear over our scrubs. Gone were the face shields that we
had to wear like helmets on our heads. Gone were the N-
95 masks. Some people were still able to find N-95 masks

to wear under their surgical masks. Those folks are quite resourceful.

The discussions today centered around not being on the COVID units. We had to re-familiarize ourselves with our home unit, including the keypad codes for locked doors behind which equipment is stored. We had gotten so accustomed to the codes on the COVID floors that it took some of us a few moments to remember the codes for our own doors. But soon, we were all back in action, answering call lights, handling various patient needs in our different corners of the unit. Not all rooms were back open. Some supplies were missing because our unit had been a ghost town for more than a month, maybe six weeks.

The odd thing about being back is that some of the patients were not the type of patients we were used to. Some were drug addicts, homeless, cardiac patients, people who had a change in mental status for some reason, and also the more familiar folks with pneumonia and difficulty breathing. You could tell that the unit was once again in transition. Our doctors were not the same ones that we're used to. It was quite a relief when I got one patient that was covered by a familiar medicine crew.

After a few hours, some of us were reminiscing about the COVID units. We felt a little guilt that we were no longer with our COVID patients. We verbalized our feelings to each other, expressing words to the effect of, "at least with COVID we knew what we were getting". This is how nursing is. We get nervous about what's coming, who's coming, we grumble about it, then we do the work.

By the time night shift came in, they too were discussing the novelty of being back on the regular unit. Someone chimed in that even if we are here today, we may be asked to go back to COVID floors on another day. A few nurses had been pulled to other floors in the hospital today. So even though we had a feeling of getting back to normal, we all knew in the backs of our minds that we weren't really back to normal, and we also were not sure

what normal is during these COVID days.

May 19th, 2020

Now that we're back on our regular unit, we do feel better about not being entrenched in the COVID units. However, COVID is far from over. Several of our patients on this floor have been transferred from the COVID units. These patients have tested negative for the virus or have been treated over several weeks and have recovered. However, some of them still have residual respiratory needs and could not be discharged home.

We still have some anxiety when it comes to former COVID patients. When we enter those rooms, we feel a bit naked without the gear we became accustomed to in the past few months. We used to have an N-95 mask, a face shield and a gown. Now, we have a surgical mask. There's something psychological about not wearing all the protection we had before. And then if the patient coughs, you have an internal panic. You imagine the droplets of something flying through the air and entering your eyes, nose or mouth. Fortunately, our noses and mouths are covered by the surgical mask, but there's no face shield to protect the eyes.

I think it will take us some time to believe that we are okay. We have to trust that the doctors safely transferred the patients from the COVID units to the regular units. We have to trust in the science that is developing at this time. It's hard to trust because there has not been much time since coronavirus disease 2019 hit us. It takes time to develop science and to experiment and to come up with verifiable findings.

Some of the nurses carried over their face shields from the COVID units. Those face shields are sanitized, of course, and stored away in lockers or backpacks. And whenever that nurse gets a patient who is a former COVID patient, out comes the trusty face shield. I'm not one of those nurses, but I do sometimes wish I had kept my face shield. Maybe I'll go back to the COVID floor and find the place where I stashed it.

Our managers announced that this week there will be a "welcome home" party for all of us who were displaced to the COVID units for several weeks. They even got a banner that attaches to the ceiling at the nurses' station that reads, "welcome home". I think that's beautiful. It gives us a sense of community, it helps us see that we are valuable nurses, and it acknowledges the sacrifices we made using our bodies to tackle COVID.

It's the day before Memorial Day, and a friend of mine invited me to a house gathering that would involve six of us. This is so normal on this weekend but there was some hesitation on my part. The city and state had not changed recommendations on gatherings but I made the decision that I would go.

I arrived wearing my home-made cloth mask and matching headband. Everyone appeared to be in good respiratory health. The host asked everyone to wash their hands as they arrived. That was a good thing on his part. As the only healthcare worker present, I had to joke around and ask everyone if they are feeling okay, if they've had any fever lately or coughing. Everyone reported that they're feeling great.

The event proceeded. The mask came off. Some of us hugged. Some of us shook hands. It was strange that doing those things which were once considered normal just didn't seem so normal anymore. But I suspect that part of recovering from COVID is getting over the psychological fears of being around other people. And also, being aware that other people could be vectors for COVID. I think we have to be willing to take some

risks, which involve leaving the comfort of your home and going to other people's homes.

The small gathering was not much different from me reporting to work. At work we wore protective equipment but when we had to eat lunch, all that equipment came off. We sat around a table and ate lunch with each other, sometimes in small groups of 4 to 6 people. We tried to social distance during those lunch meetings, but it's so hard to stay in a corner away from people who are laughing and talking. At some point it did not seem right to maintain 6 feet distance while eating lunch at work.

I hate to admit it but COVID probably loved that. That's why it's important that everyone does their part and if you feel like you're sick, you should stay away from other people. This is where we have to trust each other.

That's one of the ways we will move forward and put up a

good fight against COVID: by trusting that those of us who

may be feeling under the weather will stay home until we

feel better, thus stopping COVID from spreading from one

of us to the other.

What happens next

In the months that followed, well into the summer of 2020, COVID continued to run rampant through the United States and the world. Countries like Brazil saw thousands of people infected daily as the disease spread rapidly through the areas where poor people live. The states in the U.S. that reopened with few limits on social distancing saw huge spikes in infections. Hospitals were at capacity a few weeks after those states reopened. The governors in those states had no choice but to shut everything down again.

For us nurses, we continued to fight the fight. On the regular hospital floor, we were asked to wear surgical masks and face shields to see every patient, whether or not they were COVID positive. Every once in a while, after taking care of a patient on the regular hospital floor for a few days, a test result would come back positive and that patient had to be transferred to the COVID building where some of us had spent a few months.

We continued to wash our hands and protect

ourselves the way science told us to. We attempted to

boost our morale by coming up with an idea one day to

bring COVID-safe food to work. That meant food that was

individually packaged by a manufacturer so that no one's

hands could contaminate it, and also food such as bananas,

oranges and other citrus that could be eaten without fear of

COVID contamination.

My experience with COVID has been quite

sobering. It's a disease that turned our world upside down.

It helped us realize that capitalism is fragile. Our daily

lives in the United States of working hard then spending all

the money on our days off was paused for a while. We

learned a little more about caring for each other and staying

safe. We learned that life is not just about the stuff that you

can obtain, but it's about staying alive and showing some

love and appreciation for your family and close friends.

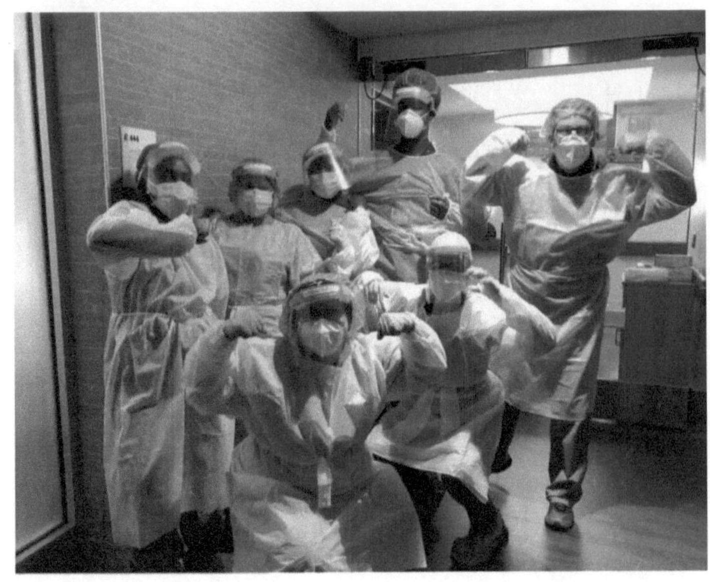

A group photo taken in the spring of 2020 showing the

strength of our COVID staff

Other books by Chad Newton

75 Mostly Gay Poems- published in 2019

Thank you

The COVID Nurse Experience

By Chad Newton

Copyright 2020